Everyd

Meals

Daily Keto Recipes to Boost your

Brain and Improve your Health.

By Luna Smith

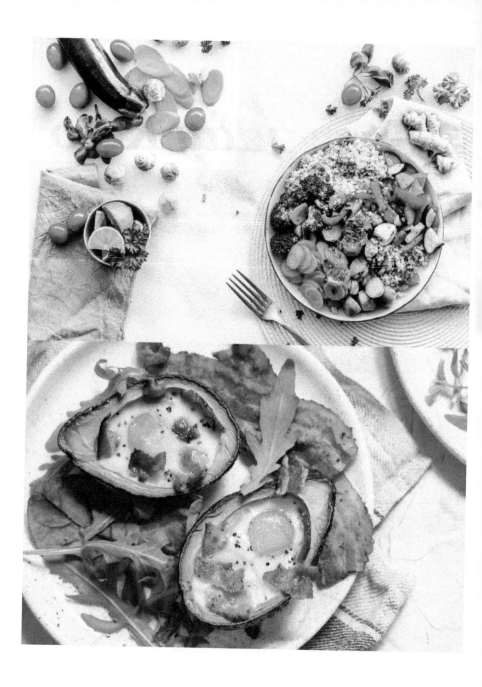

Please consult a licensed professional before attempting any techniques outlined in this book.

By reading this document, the reader agrees that under no circumstances is the author responsible for any losses, direct or indirect, which are incurred as a result of the use of information contained within this document, including, but not limited to, — errors, omissions, or inaccuracies.

Table of Contents

Shrimp Boil

Preparation Time: 15 minutes

Cooking Time: 4 hours

Servings: 4

Ingredients:

- 11/2 lb. potatoes, sliced into wedges
- 2 cloves garlic, peeled
- 2 ears corn
- 1lb. sausage, sliced
- ¼ cup Old Bay seasoning
- 1 tablespoon lemon juice
- 2 cups water
- 2lb. shrimp, peeled

Directions:

1. Put the potatoes in your slow cooker. Add the garlic, corn and sausage in layers.
2. Season with the Old Bay seasoning.
3. Drizzle lemon juice on top.
4. Pour in the water.
5. Do not mix.
6. Cover the pot.
7. Cook on high for 4 hours.
8. Add the shrimp on top.
9. Cook for 15 minutes.

Nutrition:

- Calories 585
- Fat 25.1g
- Sodium 2242mg
- Carbohydrate 3.7g
- Fiber 4.9g
- Protein 53.8g
- Sugars 3.9g

Shrimp & Sausage Gumbo

Preparation Time: 15 minutes

Cooking Time: 1 hour and 15 minutes

Servings: 4

Ingredients:

- 2 tablespoons olive oil
- 2 lb. chicken thigh fillet, sliced into cubes
- 2 cloves garlic, crushed and minced
- 1 onion, sliced
- 2 stalks celery, chopped
- 1 green bell pepper, chopped
- 1 teaspoon Cajun seasoning
- Salt to taste
- 2 cups beef broth
- 28 oz. canned crushed tomatoes
- 4 oz. sausage
- 2 tablespoons butter
- 1 lb. shrimp, peeled and deveined

Directions:

1. Pour the olive oil in a pan over medium heat.
2. Cook the garlic and chicken for 5 minutes.
3. Add the onion, celery and bell pepper.
4. Cook until tender.

5. Season with the Cajun seasoning and salt.
6. Cook for 2 minutes.
7. Stir in the sausage, broth and tomatoes.
8. Cover and cook on low for 1 hour.
9. Add the butter and shrimp in the last 10 minutes of cooking.

Nutrition:

- Calories 467
- Fat 33 g
- Sodium 1274 mg
- Carbohydrate 5 g
- Fiber 2 g
- Protein 33 g
- Sugars 5 g

Fish Stew

Preparation Time: 15 minutes

Cooking Time: 1 hour and 24 minutes

Servings: 2

- **Ingredients**
- 1 lb. white fish
- 1 tablespoon lime juice
- 1 onion, sliced
- 2 cloves garlic, sliced
- 1 red pepper, sliced
- 1 jalapeno pepper, sliced
- 1 teaspoon paprika
- 2 cups chicken broth
- 2 cups tomatoes, chopped
- Salt and pepper to taste
- 2 oz. coconut milk

Directions:

1. Marinate the fish in lime juice for 10 minutes.
2. Pour the olive oil into a pan over medium heat.
3. Add the onion, garlic and peppers.
4. Cook for 4 minutes.
5. Add the rest of the ingredients except the coconut milk.
6. Cover the pot.
7. Cook on low for 1 hour.

8. Stir in the coconut milk and simmer for 10 minutes

Nutrition:

- Calories 323
- Fat 28.6g
- Sodium 490mg
- Carbohydrate 1.1g
- Protein 9.3g
- Fiber 3.2g
- Sugars 6.2g

Salmon with Lemon & Dill

Preparation Time: 15 minutes

Cooking Time: 2 hours

Servings: 4

Ingredients:

- Cooking spray
- 1 teaspoon olive oil
- 2 lb. salmon
- 1 tablespoon fresh dill, chopped
- Salt and pepper to taste
- 1 clove garlic, minced
- 1 lemon, sliced

Directions:

1. Spray your slow cooker with oil.
2. Brush both sides of salmon with olive oil.
3. Season the salmon with salt, pepper, dill and garlic
4. Add to the slow cooker.
5. Put the lemon slices on top.
6. Cover the pot and cook on high for 2 hours.

Nutrition:

- Calories 313
- Fat 15.2g
- Sodium 102mg

- Carbohydrate 0.7g
- Fiber 0.1g
- Protein 44.2g
- Sugars 0g

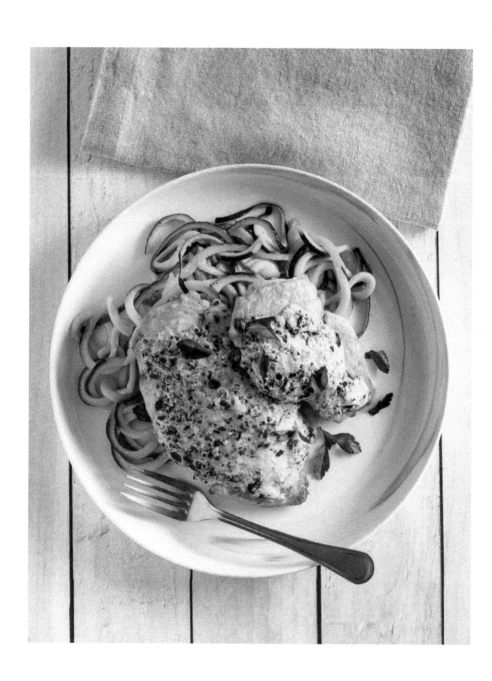

Eggs Mix

Preparation Time: 10 minutes

Cooking Time: 2 hours

Servings: 2

Ingredients:

- Cooking spray
- 3 eggs, whisked
- ¼ cup sour cream
- A pinch of salt and black pepper
- ½ teaspoon chili powder
- ½ teaspoon hot paprika
- ½ red bell pepper, chopped
- ½ yellow onion, chopped
- 3 cherry tomatoes, cubed
- 1 tablespoon parsley, chopped

Directions:

1. In a bowl, mix the eggs with the cream, salt, pepper and the other ingredients except the cooking spray and whisk well.
2. Grease your slow cooker with cooking spray, pour the eggs mix inside, spread, stir, put the lid on and cook on High for 2 hours.
3. Divide the mix between plates and serve.

Nutrition:

- Calories 162,
- Fat 5g,
- Fiber 7g
- Carbs 1.5g
- Protein 4g

Whole Seasoned Chicken

Preparation Time: 10 minutes

Cooking Time: 8 hours

Servings: 6-8

Ingredients:

- 1 large onion, cut into thick slices
- 6 garlic cloves, lightly smashed
- 1 cup chicken broth
- 3 tablespoons unsalted butter, melted
- 1 teaspoon dried rosemary
- 1 teaspoon dried sage
- 1/2 teaspoon dried thyme
- 1 teaspoon salt
- 1/4 teaspoon freshly ground black pepper
- 1 (5-pound) chicken

Directions:

1. Combine the onion, garlic, and chicken broth in the slow cooker.
2. In a small bowl, stir together the butter, rosemary, sage, thyme, salt, and pepper. Rub the spice mixture all over the chicken (make sure the chicken is dry before you do this). Place the chicken, breast-side down, on top of the onion.

3. Cover and cook on low for 8 hours, or until the thickest part of the chicken thigh reaches a temperature of 165F.

4. Carefully remove the chicken and place it on a platter or a rimmed baking sheet. Loosely tent the chicken with aluminium foil and let it rest for 10 minutes. Discard the onion, garlic, and broth.

Nutrition:

- Calories 162,
- Fat 5g,
- Fiber 7g
- Carbs 1.5g
- Protein 4g

Cheesy Barbecued Chicken Spaghetti

Preparation Time: 5 minutes

Cooking Time: 8 hours

Servings: 6-8

Ingredients:

- 2 pounds bone-in, skinless chicken thighs, trimmed of excess fat
- 2 cups tomato sauce
- ½ cup barbecue sauce
- 8 ounces angel hair pasta
- 2 cups shredded sharp Cheddar cheese

Directions:

1. Put the chicken in the slow cooker.
2. In a large bowl, mix the tomato sauce and barbecue sauce. Pour the sauce over the chicken.
3. Cover and cook on low for 8 hours.
4. Carefully transfer the chicken to a cutting board.
5. Break the angel hair pasta into 1-inch pieces. Add them to the slow cooker. Stir the sauce over the noodles. Cover and turn the slow cooker to high for 10 minutes.
6. Remove the bones and cartilage from the chicken. Shred the chicken with two forks or cut it into small pieces.

7. Once the pasta is cooked through (about 10 minutes), return the shredded chicken to the slow cooker and stir in the cheese. Scoop onto serving plates and serve.

Nutrition:

- Calories 213,
- Fat 4g,
- Fiber 8g
- Carbs 2.9g
- Protein 14g

Onion Beef

Preparation Time: 10 minutes

Cooking Time: 5 hours

Servings: 4

Ingredients:

- 4-pounds beef sirloin, sliced
- 1 teaspoon ground black pepper
- 2 cups white onion, chopped
- 1 teaspoon salt
- 2 cups of water
- 1 bay leaf
- 1/2 cup butter

Directions:

1. Mix beef sirloin with salt and ground black pepper and transfer to the slow cooker.
2. Add butter, water, onion, and bay leaf.
3. Close the lid and cook the meat on High for 5.5 hours.

Nutrition:

- Calories 176
- Fat 4 g
- Carbohydrates 1 g
- Sugar 4 g
- Protein 18

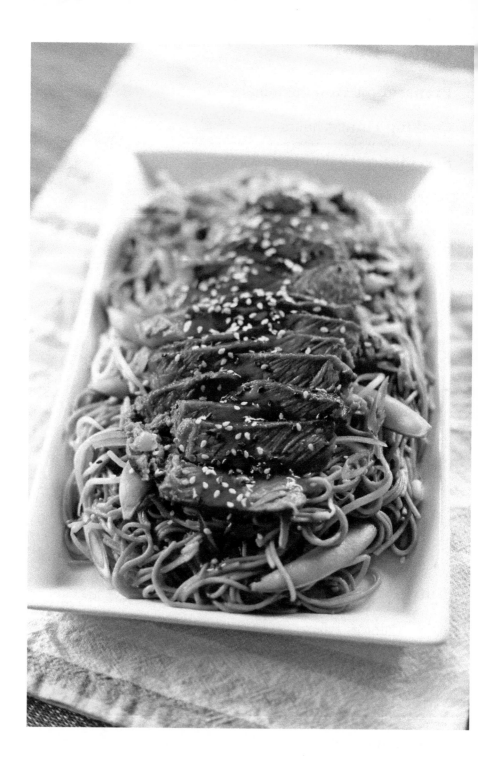

Cilantro Beef

Preparation Time: 10 minutes

Cooking Time: 4 hours

Servings: 4

Ingredients:

- 1-pound beef loin, roughly chopped
- ¼ cup apple cider vinegar
- 1 tablespoon dried cilantro
- ½ teaspoon dried basil
- 1 cup of water
- 1 teaspoon tomato paste

Directions:

1. Mix meat with tomato paste, dried cilantro, and basil.
2. Then transfer it to the slow cooker.
3. Add apple cider vinegar and water.
4. Cook the cilantro beef for 4.5 hours on High.

Nutrition:

- Calories 176
- Fat 4 g
- Carbohydrates 1 g
- Sugar 4 g
- Protein 18

Garlic Sweet Potato

Preparation Time: 10 minutes

Cooking Time: 6 hours

Servings: 4

Ingredients:

- 2-pounds sweet potatoes, chopped
- 1 teaspoon salt
- 1 teaspoon minced garlic water
- 1tablespoons vegan butter

Directions:

1. Pour water into the slow cooker. Add sweet potatoes.
2. Then add salt and close the lid.
3. Cook the sweet potato on Low for 6 hours.
4. After this, drain the water and transfer the vegetables in the big bowl.
5. Add minced garlic and butter. Carefully stir the sweet potatoes until butter is melted.

Nutrition:

- Calories 127
- Fat 3 g
- Carbohydrates 2 g
- Sugar 3 g
- Protein 21

Potato Salad

Preparation Time: 10 minutes

Cooking Time: 3 hours

Servings: 2

Ingredients:

- 1 cup potato, chopped
- 1 cup of water
- 1 teaspoon salt
- 1 oz. celery stalk, chopped
- 1 oz. fresh parsley, chopped
- ¼ onion, diced
- 1 tablespoon mayonnaise

Directions:

1. Put the potatoes in the slow cooker.
2. Add water and salt.
3. Cook the potatoes on High for 3 hours.
4. Then drain water and transfer the potatoes in the salad bowl. 5 Add all remaining ingredients and carefully mix the salad.

Nutrition:

- Calories 165
- Fat 13 g
- Carbohydrates 1.9 g

- Sugar 3 g
- Protein 28

Sautéed Greens

Preparation Time: 15 minutes

Cooking Time: 5 hours

Servings: 1

Ingredients:

- 1 cup spinach, chopped
- 2 cups water
- 1 cup collard greens, chopped
- 1/2 cup half and half
- 1 cup Swiss chard, chopped

Directions:

1. Put spinach, collard greens, and Swiss chard in the slow cooker, add water and close the lid.
2. Cook the greens on High for 1 hour.
3. Then drain water and transfer the greens in the bowl.
4. Bring the half and half to boil and pour over greens.
5. Carefully mix the greens.

Nutrition:

- Calories 112
- Fat 19 g
- Carbohydrates 1.9 g
- Sugar 3 g
- Protein 28

Slow Cooker Spaghetti Squash

Preparation Time: 15 minutes

Cooking Time: 4 hours

Servings: 5

Ingredients:

- 1-pound spaghetti squash
- 1 tablespoon butter
- 1/4 cup water
- 1 teaspoon ground black pepper
- 1/4 teaspoon ground nutmeg

Directions:

1. Peel the spaghetti squash and sprinkle it with the ground black pepper and ground nutmeg.
2. Pour water in the slow cooker.
3. Add butter and spaghetti squash.
4. Close the lid and cook for 4 hours on Low.
5. Chop the spaghetti squash into small pieces and serve!

Nutrition:

- Calories 50,
- Fat 2.9g,
- Fiber 6.6g,
- Carbs 0.1g,
- Protein 0.7g

Mushroom Stew

Preparation Time: 15 minutes

Cooking Time: 6 hours

Servings: 8

Ingredients:

- 10 oz. white mushrooms, sliced
- 2 eggplants, chopped
- 1 onion, diced
- 1 garlic clove, diced
- 2 bell peppers, chopped
- 1 cup water
- 1 tablespoon butter
- 1/2 teaspoon salt
- 1/2 teaspoon ground black pepper

Directions:

1. Place the sliced mushrooms, chopped eggplant, and diced onion into the slow cooker.
2. Add garlic clove and bell peppers.
3. Sprinkle the vegetables with salt and ground black pepper.
4. Add butter and water and stir it gently with a wooden spatula.
5. Close the lid and cook the stew for 6 hours on Low.
6. Stir the cooked stew one more time and serve!

Nutrition:

- Calories 71
- Fat 1.9g,
- Fiber 5.9g,
- Carbs 1.3g,
- Protein 3g

Cabbage Steaks

Preparation Time: 15 minutes

Cooking Time: 2 hours

Servings: 4

Ingredients:

- 10 oz. white cabbage
- 1 tablespoon butter
- 1/2 teaspoon cayenne pepper
- 1/2 teaspoon chili flakes
- 4 tablespoons water

Directions:

1. Slice the cabbage into medium steaks and rub them with the cayenne pepper and chili flakes.
2. Rub the cabbage steaks with butter on each side.
3. Place them in the slow cooker and sprinkle with water.
4. Close the lid and cook the cabbage steaks for 2 hours on High.
5. When the cabbage steaks are cooked, they should be tender to the touch.
6. Serve the cabbage steak after 10 minutes of chilling.

Nutrition:

- Calories 44,
- Fat 3g,

- Fiber 1.8g,
- Carbs 4.3g,
- Protein 1g

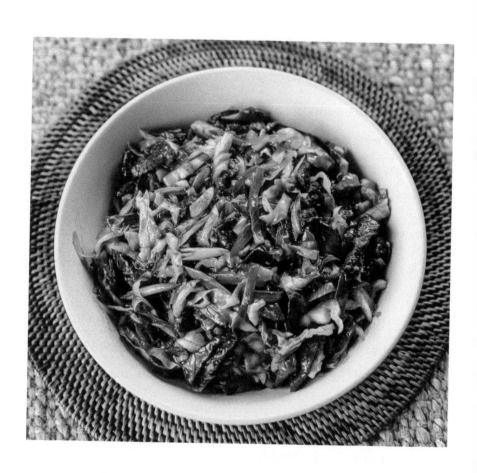

Mashed Cauliflower

Preparation Time: 20 minutes

Cooking Time: 3 hours

Servings: 5

Ingredients:

- 3 tablespoons butter
- 1-pound cauliflower
- 1 tablespoon full-fat cream
- 1 teaspoon salt
- 1 teaspoon ground black pepper
- 1 oz. dill, chopped

Directions:

1. Wash the cauliflower and chop it.
2. Place the chopped cauliflower in the slow cooker.
3. Add butter and full-fat cream.
4. Add salt and ground black pepper.
5. Stir the mixture and close the lid.
6. Cook the cauliflower for 3 hours on High.
7. When the cauliflower is cooked, transfer it to a blender and blend until smooth.
8. Place the smooth cauliflower in a bowl and mix with the chopped dill.
9. Stir it well and serve!

Nutrition:

- Calories 101,
- Fat 7.4g,
- Fiber 3.2g,
- Carbs 3.8g,
- Protein 3.1g

Bacon Wrapped Cauliflower

Preparation Time: 15 minutes

Cooking Time: 7 hours

Servings: 4

Ingredients:

- 11 oz. cauliflower head
- 3 oz. bacon, sliced
- 1 teaspoon salt
- 1 teaspoon cayenne pepper
- 1 oz. butter, softened
- 3/4 cup water

Directions:

1. Sprinkle the cauliflower head with the salt and cayenne pepper then rub with butter.
2. Wrap the cauliflower head in the sliced bacon and secure with toothpicks.
3. Pour water in the slow cooker and add the wrapped cauliflower head.
4. Cook the cauliflower head for 7 hours on Low.
5. Then let the cooked cauliflower head cool for 10 minutes.
6. Serve it!

Nutrition:

- Calories 187,

- Fat 14.8g,
- Fiber 2.1g,
- Carbs 4.7g,
- Protein 9.5g

Cauliflower Rice

Preparation Time: 15 minutes

Cooking Time: 2 hours

Servings: 5

Ingredients:

- 1-pound cauliflower
- 1 teaspoon salt
- 1 tablespoon turmeric
- 1 tablespoon butter
- 3/4 cup water

Directions:

1. Chop the cauliflower into tiny pieces to make cauliflower rice. You can also pulse in a food processor to get very fine grains of 'rice'.
2. Place the cauliflower rice in the slow cooker.
3. Add salt, turmeric, and water.
4. Stir gently and close the lid.
5. Cook the cauliflower rice for 2 hours on High.
6. Strain the cauliflower rice and transfer it to a bowl.
7. Add butter and stir gently.
8. Serve it!

Nutrition:

- Calories 48,

- Fat 2.5g,
- Fiber 2.6g,
- Carbs 5 g
- Protein 1.9g

Garlic Cauliflower Steaks

Preparation Time: 15 minutes

Cooking Time: 3 hours

Servings: 4

Ingredients:

- 14 oz. cauliflower head
- 1 teaspoon minced garlic
- 4 tablespoons butter
- 4 tablespoons water
- 1 teaspoon paprika

Directions:

1. Wash the cauliflower head carefully and slice it into the medium steaks.
2. Mix up together the butter, minced garlic, and paprika.
3. Rub the cauliflower steaks with the butter mixture.
4. Pour the water in the slow cooker.
5. Add the cauliflower steaks and close the lid.
6. Cook the vegetables for 3 hours on High.
7. Transfer the cooked cauliflower steaks to a platter and serve them immediately!

Nutrition:

- Calories 129,
- Fat 11.7g,

- Fiber 2.7g,
- Carbs 5g,
- Protein 2.2g

Zucchini Gratin

Preparation Time: 10 minutes

Cooking Time: 5 hours

Servings: 3

Ingredients:

- 1 zucchini, sliced
- 3 oz. Parmesan, grated
- 1 teaspoon ground black pepper
- 1 tablespoon butter
- 1/2 cup almond milk

Directions:

1. Sprinkle the sliced zucchini with the ground black pepper.
2. Chop the butter and place it in the slow cooker.
3. Transfer the sliced zucchini to the slow cooker to make the bottom layer.
4. Add the almond milk.
5. Sprinkle the zucchini with the grated cheese and close the lid.
6. Cook the gratin for 5 hours on Low.
7. Then let the gratin cool until room temperature.
8. Serve it!

Nutrition:

- Calories 229,
- Fat 19.6g,
- Fiber 1.8g,
- Carbs 5g,
- Protein 10.9g

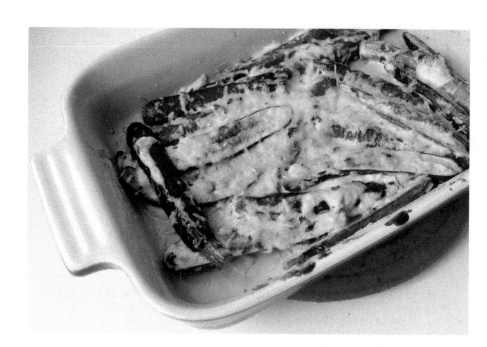

Eggplant Gratin

Preparation Time: 15 minutes

Cooking Time: 5 hours

Servings: 7

Ingredients:

- 1 tablespoon butter
- 1 teaspoon minced garlic
- 2 eggplants, chopped
- 1 teaspoon salt
- 1 tablespoon dried parsley
- 4 oz. Parmesan, grated
- 4 tablespoons water
- 1 teaspoon chili flakes

Directions:

1. Mix the dried parsley, chili flakes, and salt together.
2. Sprinkle the chopped eggplants with the spice mixture and stir well.
3. Place the eggplants in the slow cooker.
4. Add the water and minced garlic.
5. Add the butter and sprinkle with the grated Parmesan.
6. Close the lid and cook the gratin for 5 hours on Low.
7. Open the lid and cool the gratin for 10 minutes.
8. Serve it.

Nutrition:

- Calories 107,
- Fat 5.4g,
- Fiber 5.6g,
- Carbs 1.0g,
- Protein 6.8g

Broccoli and Chicken Casserole

Preparation Time: 15 minutes

Cooking Time: 35 minutes

Servings: 6

Ingredients:

- 2 tablespoons butter
- 1/4 cup cooked bacon, crumbled
- 21/2cups cheddar cheese, shredded and divided
- 4 ounces cream cheese, softened
- 1/4 cup heavy whipping cream
- ½ pack ranch seasoning mix
- 2/3 cup homemade chicken broth
- 11/2 cups small broccoli florets
- 2 cups cooked grass-fed chicken breast, shredded

Directions:

1. Preheat your oven to 350°F.
2. Arrange a rack in the upper portion of the oven.
3. For the chicken mixture: In a large wok, melt the butter over low heat.
4. Add the bacon, 1/2cup of cheddar cheese, cream cheese, heavy whipping cream, ranch seasoning, and broth, and with a wire whisk, beat until well combined.
5. Cook for about 5 minutes, stirring frequently.

6. Meanwhile, in a microwave-safe dish, place the broccoli and microwave until desired tenderness is achieved.
7. In the wok, add the chicken and broccoli and mix until well combined.
8. Remove from the heat and transfer the mixture into a casserole dish.
9. Top the chicken mixture with the remaining cheddar cheese.
10. Bake for about 25 minutes.
11. Now, set the oven to broiler.
12. Broil the chicken mixture for about 2–3 minutes or until cheese is bubbly.
13. Serve hot.

Nutrition:

- Calories: 431
- Fat: 10.5g
- Fiber: 9.1g
- Carbohydrates:4.9 g
- Protein: 14.1g

Asiago Drumsticks with Spinach

Preparation Time: 10 minutes

Cooking Time: 12minutes

Servings: 2

Ingredients:

- 1 tablespoon peanut oil
- 2 chicken drumsticks
- ½ cup vegetable broth
- ½ cup cream cheese
- 2 cups baby spinach
- Sea salt and ground black pepper, to taste
- ½ teaspoon parsley flakes
- ½ teaspoon shallot powder
- ½ teaspoon garlic powder
- ½ cup Asiago cheese, grated

Directions:

1. Heat the oil in a pan over medium-high heat. Then cook the chicken for 7 minutes, turning occasionally; reserve.

2. Pour in broth; add cream cheese and spinach; cook until spinach has wilted. Add the chicken back to the pan.

3. Add seasonings and Asiago cheese; cook until everything is thoroughly heated, an additional 4 minutes. Serve immediately and enjoy!

Nutrition:

- Calories: 588
- Fat: 46.0g
- Protein: 37.6g
- Carbs: 5.7g
- Net carbs: 4.7g
- Fiber: 1.0g

Chicken Meatloaf Cups with Pancetta

Preparation Time: 15 minutes

Cooking Time: 30 minutes

Servings: 6

Ingredients:

- 2 tbsp. onion, chopped
- 1 tsp. garlic, minced
- 1-pound ground chicken
- 2 ounces cooked pancetta, chopped
- 1 egg, beaten
- 1 tsp. mustard
- Salt and black pepper, to taste
- ½ tsp. crushed red pepper flakes
- 1 tsp. dried basil
- ½ tsp. dried oregano
- 4 ounces cheddar cheese, cubed

Directions:

1. In a mixing bowl, mix mustard, onion, ground turkey, egg, bacon, and garlic. Season with oregano, red pepper, black pepper, basil, and salt.
2. Split the mixture into muffin cups—lower one cube of cheddar cheese into each meatloaf cup.
3. Close the top to cover the cheese.

4. Bake in the oven at 345°F for 20 minutes, or until the meatloaf cups become golden brown.

Nutrition:

- Calories: 231
- Fat: 10.4g
- Fiber: 5.1g
- Carbohydrates:3.9 g
- Protein: 11.4g

Turkey Wing Curry

Preparation Time: 15 minutes

Cooking Time: 55 minutes

Servings: 4

Ingredients:

- 3 teaspoons sesame oil
- 1 pound (454 g)turkey wings, boneless and chopped
- 2 cloves garlic, finely chopped
- 1 small-sized red chili pepper, minced
- ½ teaspoon turmeric powder
- ½ teaspoon ginger powder
- 1 teaspoon red curry paste
- 1 cup unsweetened coconut milk, preferably homemade
- ½ cup water
- ½ cup turkey consommé
- Kosher salt and ground black pepper, to taste

Directions:

1. Heat sesame oil in a sauté pan. Add the turkey and cook until it is light brown about 7 minutes.

2. Add garlic, chili pepper, turmeric powder, ginger powder, and curry paste and cook for 3 minutes longer.

3. Add the milk, water, and consommé. Season with salt and black pepper. Cook for 45 minutes over medium heat. Bon appétit!

Nutrition:

- Calories: 296
- Fat: 19.6g
- Protein: 25.6g
- Carbs: 3.0g
- Net carbs: 3.0g
- Fiber: 0g

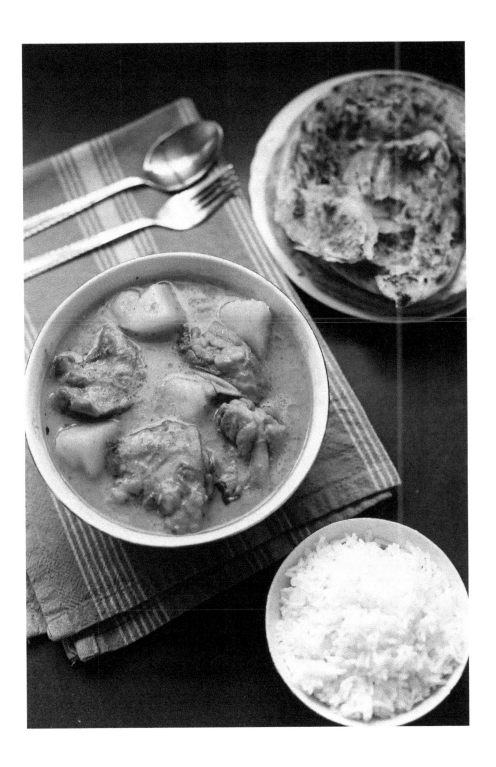

Double-Cheese Ranch Chicken

Preparation Time: 15 minutes

Cooking Time: 20 minutes

Servings: 4

Ingredients:

- 2 chicken breasts
- 2 tablespoons butter, melted
- 1 teaspoon salt
- ½ teaspoon garlic powder
- ½ teaspoon cayenne pepper
- ½ teaspoon black peppercorns, crushed
- ½ tablespoon ranch seasoning mix
- 4 ounces (113 g) Ricotta cheese, room temperature
- ½ cup Monterey-Jack cheese, grated
- 4 slices bacon, chopped
- ¼ cup scallions, chopped

Directions:

1. Start by preheating your oven to 370°F (188°C).

2. Drizzle the chicken with melted butter. Rub the chicken with salt, garlic powder, cayenne pepper, black pepper, and ranch seasoning mix.

3. Heat a cast iron skillet over medium heat. Cook the chicken for 3 to 5 minutes per side. Transfer the chicken to a lightly greased baking dish.

4. Add cheese and bacon. Bake about 12minutes. Top with scallions just before serving. Bon appétit!

Nutrition:

- Calories: 290
- Fat: 19.3g
- Protein: 25.1g
- Carbs: 2.5g
- Net carbs: 2.5g
- Fiber: 0g

Turkey and Canadian Bacon Pizza

Preparation Time: 10 minutes

Cooking Time: 32minutes

Servings: 4

Ingredients:

- ½ pound (227 g) ground turkey
- ½ cup Parmesan cheese, freshly grated
- ½ cup Mozzarella cheese, grated
- Salt and ground black pepper, to taste
- 1 bell pepper, sliced
- 2 slices Canadian bacon, chopped
- 1 tomato, chopped
- 1 teaspoon oregano
- ½ teaspoon basil

Directions:

1. In mixing bowl, thoroughly combine the ground turkey, cheese, salt, and black pepper.

2. Then, press the cheese-chicken mixture into a parchment-lined baking pan. Bake in the preheated oven, at 390°F (199°C) for 22minutes.

3. Add bell pepper, bacon, tomato, oregano, and basil. Bake an additional 10 minutes and serve warm. Bon appétit!

Nutrition:

- Calories: 361
- Fat: 22.6g
- Protein: 32.5g
- Carbs: 5.8g
- Net carbs: 5.2g
- Fiber: 0.6g

Grilled Rosemary Wings with Leeks

Preparation Time: 10 minutes

Cooking Time: 20 minutes

Servings: 4

Ingredients:

- 8 chicken wings
- 2 tablespoons butter, melted The Marinade:
- 2 garlic cloves, minced
- ¼ cup leeks, chopped
- 2 tablespoons lemon juice
- Salt and ground black pepper, to taste
- ½ teaspoon paprika
- 1 teaspoon dried rosemary

Directions:

1. Thoroughly combine all ingredients for the marinade in a ceramic bowl. Add the chicken wings to the bowl.

2. Cover and allow it to marinate for 1hour.

3. Then, preheat your grill to medium-high heat. Drizzle melted butter over the chicken wings. Grill the chicken wings for 20 minutes, turning them periodically.

4. Taste, adjust the seasonings, and serve warm. Enjoy!

Nutrition:

- Calories: 132
- Fat: 7.9g
- Protein: 13.3g
- Carbs: 1.9g
- Net carbs: 1.6g
- Fiber: 0.3g

Buffalo Chicken Bake

Preparation Time: 10 minutes

Cooking Time: 55 minutes

Servings: 6

Ingredients:

- 1 tablespoon olive oil
- 2 pounds (907 g) chicken drumettes
- Sauce:
- ½ cup melted butter
- ½ cup hot sauce
- 2 tablespoons white vinegar
- ¼ teaspoon granulated garlic
- Sea salt and ground black, to season

Directions:

1. Start by preheating your oven to 320°F (160°C). Brush a baking pan with olive oil. Arrange the chicken drumettes in the greased pan.

2. Prepare the sauce by whisking the melted butter, hot sauce, white vinegar, garlic, salt and black pepper until well combined.

3. Pour the sauce over the chicken drumettes. Bake for 55 minutes, flipping the chicken drumettes once or twice.

4. Taste, adjust the seasonings and serve warm.

Nutrition:

- Calories: 289
- Fat: 20.5g
- Protein: 23.4g
- Carbs: 1.3g
- Net carbs: 1.0g
- Fiber: 0.3g

Chinese Flavor Chicken Legs

Preparation Time: 10 minutes

Cooking Time: 15 minutes

Servings: 4

Ingredients:

- 1 tablespoon sesame oil
- 4 chicken legs
- ¼ cup Shaoxing wine
- 2 tablespoons brown erythritol
- ¼ cup spicy tomato sauce

Directions:

1. Heat the sesame oil in a cast-iron skillet over medium-high flame. Now, sear chicken wings until they turn golden in color on all sides; reserve.

2. Then, in the same skillet, add a splash of wine to deglaze the pan.

3. Add in the remaining wine, brown erythritol, and spicy tomato sauce. Bring to a boil and immediately reduce the heat to medium-low.

4. Let it simmer for 5 to 10 minutes until the sauce coats the back of a spoon. Add the reserved chicken legs back to the skillet.

5. Cook for a further 3 minutes or until the chicken is well coated and heated through. Enjoy!

Nutrition:

- Calories: 366
- Fat: 14.6g
- Protein: 51.1g
- Carbs: 3.4g
- Net carbs: 2.4g
- Fiber: 1.0g

Cheesy Brussels Sprouts and Eggs

Preparation Time: 5 minutes

Cooking Time: 20 minutes

Servings: 4

Ingredients:

- 1 tablespoon olive oil
- 1 pound Brussels sprouts, shredded
- 4 eggs, whisked
- ½-cup coconut cream
- Salt and black pepper to the taste
- 1 tablespoon chives, chopped
- ¼ cup cheddar cheese, shredded

Directions:

1. Preheat the Air Fryer at 360 degrees F and grease it with the oil.
2. Spread the Brussels sprouts on the bottom of the fryer, then add the eggs mixed with the rest of the ingredients, toss a bit and cook for 20 minutes.
3. Divide between plates and serve.

Nutrition:

- Calories 242

- Fat 12g
- Fiber 3g
- Carbohydrates 5g
- Protein 9g

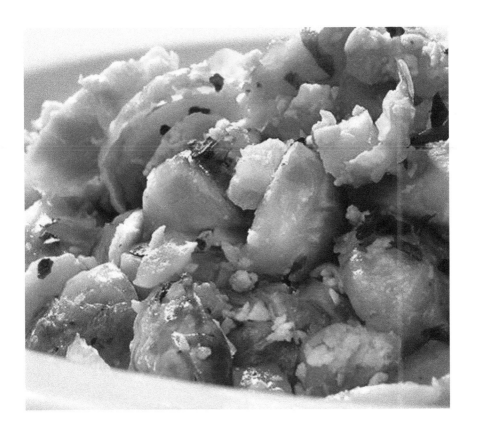

Savory Ham and Cheese Waffles

Preparation Time: 10 minutes

Cooking Time: 10 minutes

Servings: 2

Ingredients:

- 2 ounces (57 g) ham steak, chopped
- 2 ounces (57 g) Cheddar cheese, grated
- 8 eggs
- 1 teaspoon baking powder
- Basil, to taste
- From the cupboard:
- 12 tablespoons butter, melted
- Olive oil, as needed
- 1-teaspoon sea salt
- Special Equipment:
- A waffle iron

Directions:

1. Preheat the waffle iron and set aside.
2. Crack the eggs and keep the egg yolks and egg whites in two separate bowls.
3. Add the butter, baking powder, basil, and salt to the egg yolks. Whisk well. Fold in the chopped ham and stir until well combined. Set aside.

4. Lightly season the egg whites with salt and beat until it forms stiff peaks.
5. Add the egg whites into the bowl of egg yolk mixture. Allow to sit for about 5 minutes.
6. Lightly coat the waffle iron with the olive oil. Slowly pour half of the mixture in the waffle iron and cook for about 4 minutes. Repeat with the remaining egg mixture.
7. Take off from the waffle iron and serve warm on two serving plates.

Nutrition:

- Calories: 636
- Fat: 50.2g
- Protein: 45.1g
- Net carbs: 1.1g

Classic Spanakopita Frittata

Preparation Time: 10 minutes

Cooking Time: 3-4 hours

Servings: 8

Ingredients:

- 12 eggs, beaten
- ½ cup feta cheese
- 1 cup heavy whipping cream
- 2 cups spinach, chopped
- 2 teaspoons garlic, minced
- From the cupboard:
- 1 tablespoon extra-virgin olive oil

Directions:

1. Grease the bottom of the slow cooker, put with the olive oil lightly.
2. Stir together the beaten eggs, feta cheese, heavy cream, spinach, and garlic until well combined.
3. Slowly pour the mixture into the slow cooker. Cook covered on LOW for 3 to 4 hours, or until a knife inserted in the center comes out clean.
4. Take off from the slow cooker and cool for about 3 minutes before slicing.

Nutrition:

- Calories: 254
- Fat: 22.3g
- Protein: 11.1g
- Net carbs: 2.1g
- Fiber: 0g
- Cholesterol: 364mg

Sausage Stuffed Bell Peppers

Preparation Time: 15 minutes

Cooking Time: 4-5 hours

Servings: 4

Ingredients:

- 1 cup breakfast sausage, crumbled
- 4 bell peppers, seedless and cut the top
- ½ cup coconut milk
- 6 eggs
- 1 cup cheddar cheese, shredded
- From the cupboard:
- 1 tablespoon extra-virgin olive oil
- ½ teaspoon freshly ground black pepper

Directions:

1. Add the coconut milk, eggs, and black pepper in a medium bowl, whisking until smooth. Set aside.
2. Line your slow cooker inserts with aluminium foil. Grease the aluminium foil with 1 tablespoon olive oil.
3. Evenly stuff four bell peppers with the crumbled sausage and spoon the egg mixture into the peppers.
4. Arrange the stuffed peppers in the slow cooker. Sprinkle the cheese on top.
5. Cook covered on LOW for 4 to 5 hours, or until the peppers are browned and the eggs are completely set.

6. Divide in 4 serving plates and serve warm.

Nutrition:

- Calories: 459
- Fat: 36.3g
- Protein: 25.2g
- Net carbs: 7.9g
- Fiber: 3g
- Cholesterol: 376mg

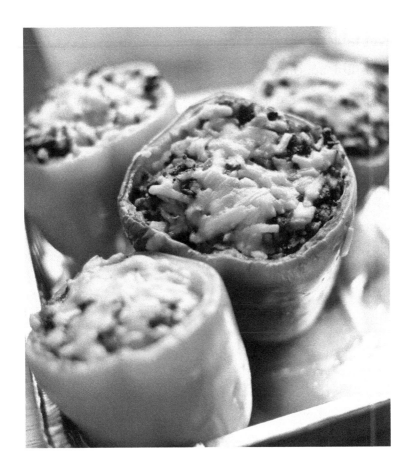

Homemade Sausage, Egg, and Cheese Sandwich

Preparation Time: 5 minutes

Cooking Time: 30 minutes

Servings: 1

Ingredients:

Muffin:

- 1 egg
- 1 tablespoon coconut flour
- 1 tablespoon almond milk
- ½ tablespoon olive oil
- ½-teaspoon baking powder
- Pinch of salt

Filling:

- 1 egg
- ¼-pound breakfast sausage
- 1 slice cheddar cheese

Directions:

1. Preheat oven to 400-degrees.
2. Begin by mixing your muffin batter together first by cracking an egg in a bowl, then mixing in the rest of the ingredients.
3. Grease a ramekin and pour in the batter.

4. Bake for 15 minutes.

5. To get an egg that's the same size as your muffin, crack an egg in a ramekin and whisk.

6. Flavor with salt and pepper, then bake for 10 minutes.

7. For your sausage, just form the meat into a patty.

8. Heat a skillet, and then cook patty for 4-5 minutes per side.

9. When the muffins are ready, remove from oven and carefully slice in half.

10. For a toasty muffin, stick in a toaster for a few minutes.

11. Build sandwich and top with a slice of cheese.

12. Eat!

Nutrition:

- Calories: 460
- Protein: 29g
- Carbs: 3g
- Fat: 37g
- Fiber: 0g

Chicken Sausage Breakfast Casserole

Preparation Time: 10 minutes

Cooking Time: 40 minutes

Servings: 4

Ingredients:

- 1 pound chicken sausage
- 3 big eggs
- 2 cups chopped tomatoes
- 2 cups diced zucchini
- 1 ½ cups cheddar cheese
- ½ cup diced onion
- ½ cup plain Greek yogurt
- 1 teaspoon dried sage
- 1 teaspoon dried mustard

Directions:

1. Preheat oven to 375-degrees.
2. Preheat a skillet until warm, then add sausage.
3. When nearly all the pink is gone, put the zucchini and onion.
4. Cook until the veggies are softened.
5. Move skillet contents to a greased casserole dish.
6. In a separate bowl, mix eggs, yogurt, and seasonings together.
7. Lastly, mix one cup of cheese into eggs.

8. Pour into the casserole dish on top of the sausage and veggies.
9. Bake for at least 30 minutes until cheese has melted and starts browning.
10. Serve right away!

Nutrition:

- Calories: 487
- Protein: 19g
- Carbs: 4.8g
- Fat: 42g
- Fiber: 1.3g

Cheddar-Chive Omelet for One

Preparation Time: 8 minutes

Cooking Time: 5 minutes

Servings: 1

Ingredients:

- 2 slices cooked bacon
- 2 big eggs
- 2 stalks chives
- 2 tablespoons sharp cheddar cheese
- 1 teaspoon olive oil
- Salt and pepper to taste

Directions:

1. Heat oil in a skillet.
2. While that heats, chop chives.
3. Pour in eggs and sprinkle chives, salt, and pepper on top.
4. Wait until edges are beginning to set.
5. Crumble bacon on top and wait another 25 seconds.
6. Remove skillet from heat.
7. Sprinkle on cheese and carefully fold omelet over.
8. Enjoy!

Nutrition:

- Calories: 463
- Protein: 24g

- Carbs: 1g
- Fat: 39g
- Fiber: 1g

Lunch Chicken Wraps

Preparation Time: 18 minutes

Cooking Time: 6 hours

Servings: 6

Ingredients:

- 6 tortillas
- 3 tablespoon Caesar dressing
- 1-pound chicken breast
- 1/2 cup lettuce
- 1 cup water
- 1 oz. bay leaf
- 1 teaspoon salt
- 1 teaspoon ground pepper
- 1 teaspoon coriander
- 4 oz. Feta cheese

Directions:

1. Put the chicken breast in the slow cooker.
2. Sprinkle the meat with the bay leaf, salt, ground pepper, and coriander.
3. Add water and cook the chicken breast for 6 hours on LOW.
4. Then remove the cooked chicken from the slow cooker and shred it with a fork.

5. Chop the lettuce roughly.

6. Then chop Feta cheese. Combine the chopped Ingredients: together and add the shredded chicken breast and Caesar dressing.

7. Mix everything together well. After this, spread the tortillas with the shredded chicken mixture and wrap them. Enjoy!

Nutrition:

- Calories 376
- Fat 18.5g
- Fiber 3g
- Carbs 2.3g
- Protein 23g

Nutritious Lunch Wraps

Preparation Time: 20 minutes

Cooking Time: 4 hours

Servings: 5

Ingredients:

- 7 oz. ground pork
- 5 tortillas
- 1 tablespoon tomato paste
- 1/2 cup onion, chopped
- 1/2 cup lettuce
- 1 teaspoon ground black pepper
- 1 teaspoon salt
- 1 teaspoon sour cream
- 5 tablespoons water
- 4 oz. Parmesan, shredded
- 2 tomatoes

Directions:

1. Combine the ground pork with the tomato paste, ground black pepper, salt, and sour cream. Transfer the meat mixture to the slow cooker and cook on HIGH for 4 hours.
2. Meanwhile, chop the lettuce roughly. Slice the tomatoes.

3. Place the sliced tomatoes in the tortillas and add the chopped lettuce and shredded Parmesan. When the ground pork is cooked, chill to room temperature.
4. Add the ground pork in the tortillas and wrap them. Enjoy!

Nutrition:

- Calories 318,
- Fat 7g,
- Fiber 2g,
- Carbs 3.76g,
- Protein 26g

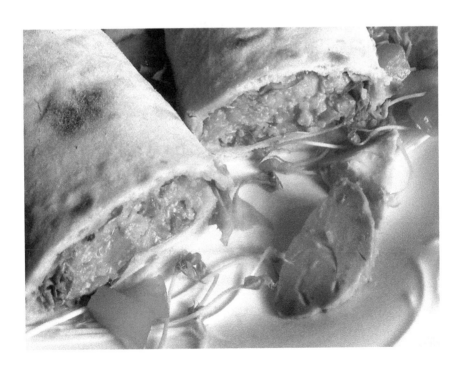

Butternut Squash Soup

Preparation Time: 10 minutes

Cooking Time: 8 hours

Servings: 9

Ingredients:

- 2-pound butternut squash
- 4 teaspoon minced garlic
- 1/2 cup onion, chopped
- ½ teaspoon salt
- 1/4 teaspoon ground nutmeg
- 1 teaspoon ground black pepper
- 8 cups chicken stock
- 1 tablespoon fresh parsley

Directions:

1. Peel the butternut squash and cut it into the chunks.
2. Toss the butternut squash in the slow cooker.
3. Add chopped onion, minced garlic, and chicken stock.
4. Close the slow cooker lid and cook the soup for 8 hours on LOW.
5. Meanwhile, combine the ground black pepper, ground nutmeg, and salt together.
6. Chop the fresh parsley.

7. When the time is done, remove the soup from the slow cooker and blend it with a blender until you get a creamy soup.

8. Sprinkle the soup with the spice mixture and add chopped parsley. Serve the soup warm. Enjoy!

Nutrition:

- Calories 129
- Fat 2.7g
- Fiber 2g
- Carbs 2.85g
- Protein 7g

Eggplant Bacon Wraps

Preparation Time: 17 minutes

Cooking Time: 5 hours

Servings: 6

Ingredients:

- 10 oz. eggplant, sliced into rounds
- 5 oz. halloumi cheese
- 1 teaspoon minced garlic
- 3 oz. bacon, chopped
- 1/2 teaspoon ground black pepper
- 1 teaspoon salt
- 1 teaspoon paprika
- 1 tomato

Directions:

1. Rub the eggplant slices with the ground black pepper, salt, and paprika.
2. Slice halloumi cheese and tomato.
3. Combine the chopped bacon and minced garlic together.
4. Place the sliced eggplants in the slow cooker. Cook the eggplant on HIGH for 1 hour.
5. Chill the eggplant. Place the sliced tomato and cheese on the eggplant slices.
6. Add the chopped bacon mixture and roll up tightly.

7. Secure the eggplants with the toothpicks and return the eggplant wraps back into the slow cookies. Cook the dish on HIGH for 4 hours more.
8. When the dish is done, serve it immediately. Enjoy!

Nutrition:

- Calories 131,
- Fat 9.4g,
- Fiber 2g,
- Carbs 1.25g,
- Protein 6 g

Mexican Warm Salad

Preparation Time: 26 minutes

Cooking Time: 10 hours

Servings: 10

Ingredients:

- 1 cup black beans
- 1 cup sweet corn, frozen
- 3 tomatoes
- 1/2 cup fresh dill
- ½ teaspoon chili pepper
- 7 oz. chicken fillet
- 5 oz. Cheddar cheese
- 4 tablespoons mayonnaise
- 1 teaspoon minced garlic
- 1 cup lettuce
- 5 cups chicken stock
- 1 cucumber

Directions:

1. Put the chicken fillet, sweet corn, black beans, and chicken stock in the slow cooker.
2. Close the slow cooker lid and cook the mixture on LOW for 10 hours.

3. When the time is done remove the mixture from the slow cooker.
4. Shred the chicken fillet with 2 forks. Chill the mixture until room temperature.
5. Chop the lettuce roughly. Chop the cucumber and tomatoes.
6. Place the lettuce, cucumber, and tomatoes on a large serving plate.
7. After this, shred Cheddar cheese and chop the chili pepper.
8. Add the chili pepper to the serving plate too.
9. After this, add the chicken mixture on the top of the salad.
10. Sprinkle the salad with the mayonnaise, minced garlic, and shredded cheese. Enjoy the salad immediately.

Nutrition:

- Calories 182,
- Fat 7.8g,
- Fiber 2g,
- Carbs 1.6g,
- Protein 9g

Hot Chorizo Salad

Preparation Time: 20 minutes

Cooking Time: 4 hours 30 minutes

Servings: 6

Ingredients:

- 8 oz. chorizo
- 1 teaspoon olive oil
- 1 teaspoon cayenne pepper
- 1 teaspoon chili flakes
- 1 teaspoon ground black pepper
- 1 teaspoon onion powder
- 2 garlic cloves
- 3 tomatoes
- 1 cup lettuce
- 1 cup fresh dill
- 1 teaspoon oregano
- 3 tablespoons crushed cashews

Directions:

1. Chop the chorizo sausages roughly and place them in the slow cooker.
2. Cook the sausages for 4 hours on HIGH.

3. Meanwhile, combine the cayenne pepper, chili flakes, ground black pepper, and onion powder together in a shallow bowl.
4. Chop the tomatoes roughly and add them to the slow cooker after 4 hours. Cook the mixture for 30 minutes more on HIGH.
5. Chop the fresh dill and combine it with oregano.
6. When the chorizo sausage mixture is cooked, place it in a serving bowl. Tear the lettuce and add it in the bowl too.
7. After this, peel the garlic cloves and slice them.
8. Add the sliced garlic cloves in the salad bowl too.
9. Then sprinkle the salad with the spice mixture, olive oil, fresh dill mixture, and crush cashew. Mix the salad carefully. Enjoy!

Nutrition:

- Calories 249,
- Fat 19.8g,
- Fiber 2g,
- Carbs 1.69g,
- Protein 11g

Chicken Fajitas

Preparation Time: 10 minutes

Cooking Time: 3 hours

Servings: 6

Ingredients:

- 11/2 lb. chicken breast fillet
- ½ cup salsa
- 2oz. cream cheese
- 1 teaspoon cumin
- 1 teaspoon paprika
- Salt and pepper to taste
- 1 onion, sliced
- 1 clove garlic, minced
- 1 red bell pepper, sliced
- 1 green bell pepper, sliced
- 1 teaspoon lime juice

Directions:

1. Combine all the ingredients except the lime wedges in your slow cooker.
2. Cover the pot.
3. Cook on high for 3 hours.
4. Shred the chicken.
5. Drizzle with lime juice.

6. Serve with toppings like sour cream and cheese.

Nutrition:

- Calories 276
- Fat 17 g
- Cholesterol 105 mg
- Sodium 827 mg
- Carbohydrate 3 g
- Protein 25 g
- Sugars 2 g

Tuscan Garlic Chicken

Preparation Time: 15 minutes

Cooking Time: 3 hours

Servings: 6

Ingredients:

- 1 tablespoon olive oil
- 2cloves garlic, crushed and minced
- ½ cup chicken broth
- 1 cup heavy cream
- ¾ cup Parmesan cheese, grated
- 2 chicken breasts
- 1 tablespoon Italian seasoning
- Salt and pepper to taste
- 1/2 cup sundried tomatoes, chopped
- 2 cups spinach, chopped

Directions:

1. Pour the oil into your pan over medium heat.
2. Cook the garlic for 1 minute.
3. Stir in the broth and cream.
4. Simmer for 10 minutes.
5. Stir in the Parmesan cheese and remove from heat.
6. Put the chicken in your slow cooker.
7. Season with the salt, pepper and Italian seasoning.

8. Place the tomatoes on top of the chicken.

9. Pour the cream mixture on top of the chicken.

10. Cover the pot.

11. Cook on high for 3 hours.

12. Take the chicken out of the slow cooker and set aside

13. Add the spinach and stir until wilted.

14. Pour the sauce over the chicken and serve with the sun-dried tomatoes and spinach.

Nutrition:

- Calories 306
- Fat 18.4g
- Cholesterol 115mg
- Sodium 287mg
- Carbohydrate 4.9g
- Protein 30.1g
- Sugars 2g

Sesame Ginger Chicken

Preparation Time: 5 minutes

Cooking Time: 5 hours

Servings: 4

Ingredients:

- 11/2 lb. chicken breast fillet
- ½ cup tomato sauce
- ¼ cup low-sugar peach jam
- ¼ cup chicken broth
- 2 tablespoons coconut amino
- 11/2 tablespoons sesame oil
- 1 tablespoon honey
- 1 teaspoon ground ginger
- 2 cloves garlic, minced
- ¼ cup onion, minced
- ¼ teaspoon red pepper flakes, crushed
- 2 tablespoons red bell pepper, chopped
- 11/2 tablespoons green onion, chopped
- 2 teaspoons sesame seeds

Directions:

1. Combine all the ingredients except green onion and sesame seeds in your slow cooker.
2. Mix well.

3. Cover the pot and cook on high for 4 hours.

4. Garnish with the green onion and sesame seeds.

Nutrition:

- Calories 220
- Fat 13 g
- Sodium 246 mg
- Carbohydrate 7 g
- Protein 26 g
- Sugars 2 g

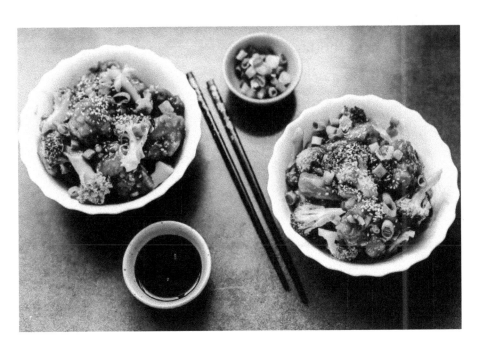

Ranch Chicken

Preparation Time: 5 minutes

Cooking Time: 4 hours and 5 minutes

Servings: 6

Ingredients:

- 2 lb. chicken breast fillet
- 2 tablespoons butter
- 2 oz. cream cheese
- 3 tablespoons ranch dressing mix

Directions:

1. Add the chicken to your slow cooker.
2. Place the butter and cream cheese on top of the chicken.
3. Sprinkle ranch dressing mix.
4. Seal the pot.
5. Cook on high for 4 hours.
6. Shred the chicken using forks and serve.

Nutrition:

- Calories 266
- Fat 12.9 g
- Sodium 167 mg
- Carbohydrate 4 g
- Fiber 0 g
- Protein 33 g

Mahi Taco Wraps

Preparation Time: 5 minutes

Cooking Time: 2 hours

Servings: 6

Ingredients:

- 1 pound Mahi Mahi, wild-caught
- 1/2 cup cherry tomatoes
- 1 small green bell pepper, cored and sliced
- 1/4 of a medium red onion, thinly sliced
- 1/2 teaspoon garlic powder
- 1 teaspoon sea salt
- 1/2 teaspoon ground black pepper
- 1 teaspoon chipotle pepper
- 1/2 teaspoon dried oregano
- 1 teaspoon cumin
- 1 tablespoon avocado oil
- 1/4 cup chicken stock
- 1 medium avocado, diced
- 1 cup sour cream
- 6 large lettuce leaves

Directions:

1. Grease a 6-quarts slow cooker with oil, place fish in it and then pour in chicken stock.

2. Stir together garlic powder, salt, black pepper, chipotle pepper, oregano and cumin and then season fish with half of this mixture.

3. Layer fish with tomatoes, pepper and onion, season with remaining spice mixture and shut with lid.

4. Plug in the slow cooker and cook fish for 2 hours at high heat setting or until cooked through.

5. When done, evenly spoon fish among lettuce, top with avocado and sour cream and serve.

Nutrition:

- Calories: 260
- Fat: 15.1 g
- Protein: 27.8 g
- Carbs: 1.9 g
- Fiber: 2.2 g
- Sugar: 3

Shrimp Tacos

Preparation Time: 5 minutes

Cooking Time: 3 hours

Servings: 6

Ingredients:

- 1 pound medium wild-caught shrimp, peeled and tails off
- 12-ounce fire-roasted tomatoes, diced
- 1 small green bell pepper, chopped
- ½ cup chopped white onion
- 1 teaspoon minced garlic
- ½ teaspoon sea salt
- ½ teaspoon ground black pepper
- ½ teaspoon red chili powder
- ½ teaspoon cumin
- 1/4 teaspoon cayenne pepper
- 2 tablespoons avocado oil
- ½ cup salsa
- 4 tablespoons chopped cilantro
- 11/2 cup sour cream
- 2 medium avocado, diced

Directions:

1. Rinse shrimps, layer into a 6-quarts slow cooker and drizzle with oil.

2. Add tomatoes, stir until mixed, then add peppers and remaining ingredients except for sour cream and avocado and stir until combined.

3. Plug in the slow cooker, shut with lid and cook for 2 to 3 hours at low heat setting or 1 hour and 30 minutes to 2 hours at high heat setting or until shrimps turn pink.

4. When done, serve shrimps with avocado and sour cream.

Nutrition:

- Calories: 324
- Fat: 12 g
- Protein: 28 g
- Carbs: 4.2 g
- Fiber: 13 g
- Sugar: 2g

Fish Curry

Preparation Time: 5 minutes

Cooking Time: 4 hours

Servings: 6

Ingredients:

- 2.2 pounds wild-caught white fish fillet, cubed
- 18-ounce spinach leaves
- 4 tablespoons red curry paste, organic
- 14-ounce coconut cream, unsweetened and full-fat
- 14-ounce water

Directions:

1. Plug in a 6-quart slow cooker and let preheat at high heat setting.
2. In the meantime, whisk together coconut cream and water until smooth.
3. Place fish into the slow cooker, spread with curry paste and then pour in coconut cream mixture.
4. Shut with lid and cook for 2 hours at high heat setting or 4 hours at low heat setting until tender.
5. Then add spinach and continue cooking for 20 to 30 minutes or until spinach leaves wilt.
6. Serve straightaway.

Nutrition:

- Calories: 129
- Fat: 6 g
- Protein: 12 g
- Carbs: 4.8 g
- Fiber: 10 g
- Sugar: 6g